YOUR KNOWLEDGE HAS VALUE

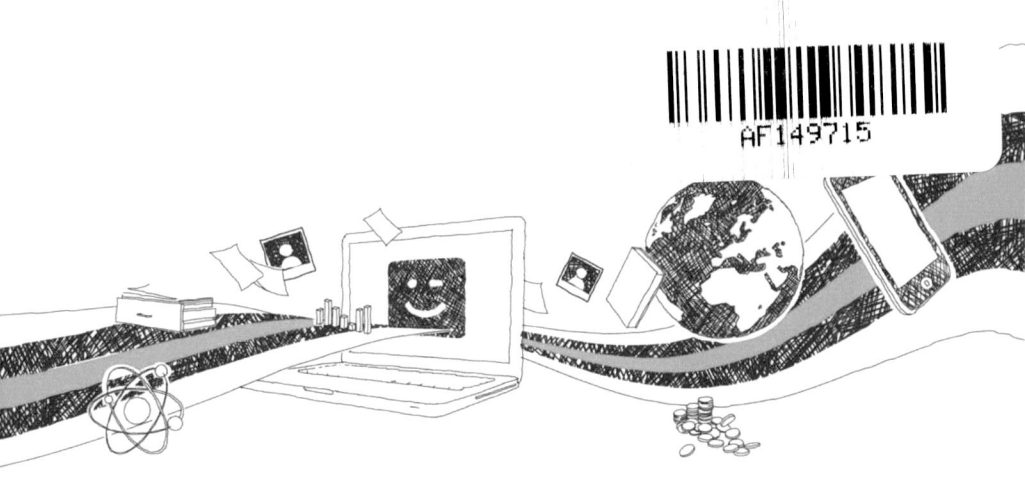
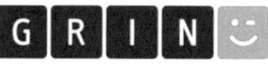

Abdalla Ibrahim

Ebola. Black death of the 21st century

Analyse of the Ebola epidemic 2014

GRIN Publishing

Bibliographic information published by the German National Library:

The German National Library lists this publication in the National Bibliography; detailed bibliographic data are available on the Internet at http://dnb.dnb.de .

Imprint:

Copyright © 2014 GRIN Verlag GmbH
Print and binding: Books on Demand GmbH, Norderstedt Germany
ISBN: 978-3-656-83730-5

This book at GRIN:

http://www.grin.com/en/e-book/283800/ebola-black-death-of-the-21st-century

GRIN - Your knowledge has value

Since its foundation in 1998, GRIN has specialized in publishing academic texts by students, college teachers and other academics as e-book and printed book. The website www.grin.com is an ideal platform for presenting term papers, final papers, scientific essays, dissertations and specialist books.

Visit us on the internet:

http://www.grin.com/

http://www.facebook.com/grincom

http://www.twitter.com/grin_com

Ebola: is it to be the black death of the 21st century?

"Analysis of Ebola epidemic 2014"

Abdalla Ibrahim, October 2014.

Introduction

Ebola is a viral disease caused by several viruses and the disease is known as Ebola hemorrhagic fever. Humans are not the natural host for it and can not be carriers. Infection is contracted by contact with carrier animals in different ways. Humans become infectious during the sickness period especially in crowded places and where culture embraces close body contact with family and friends as the disease spreads by body fluids. Generally Ebola is not a disease that might lead to an epidemic due to several reasons, the fact that there are no human carriers, the replication time of the Ebola virus makes its transmission rate limited to 1.8% and normally it kills the host before it spreads. What led to this epidemic becoming the largest of Ebola is the question to answer (PHMS, 2014).

Sierra Leone is a small country located in West Africa. Inhabitants are estimated to be around 6 million by the united nations in 2012. In terms of human development, Sierra Leone is ranked 183rd in the Human Development report (HDI) among 187 countries included, in other words, one the worst countries ranked (UNDP, 2013). Health system within Sierra Leone is not well-structured and with high out-of-pocket expenditure, life expectancy on the other hand is one of the lowest worldwide with 45.3 years at birth (World Bank database, 2013). Poverty in Sierra Leone pushed people to work in the agricultural investments, as they have huge rainforest and Savannah which allowed more contact with the host animals -mostly fruit bats- and led to the spread of disease within that slice of community at the beginning (PHMS, 2014).

Globalization and Ebola

We live in a time in which issues needed to be dealt with are not limited to one area, have growing intensity and extensity in relation to crossing geographical borders, yet the collective approaches to solve them are weak and incomplete, with the difficulties encountered are mainly due to the anemic problem-solving capacities at global and regional levels, mostly due to structural complexity that hinders urgent responses and policy-setting in reaction to global emergencies (Held, D., 2008). The lack of ownership of problems at global level, for example now after the Ebola outbreak the WHO stated that "it is technical body, and the responsibility lies first on the countries to protect their citizens", yet they are not the ones to blame. All of this is mainly due to lack of clear global governance structure, "a ship with more than a leader sinks" (Gostin, L. O., & Friedman, E. A., (2014). On the contrary, countries in which the epidemic has started are poor, and the life expectancy at birth is considered to be of the lowest worldwide, this indeed reflects the poor health status in general and the health care system within, which means that the governments aren't taking their "assumed role" as mentioned by the WHO, and if we are to improve the social determinants of health, governments of those countries must assume their role and take action in population protection and human rights provision including health (Gostin, L. O., & Friedman, E. A. 2014).

The world has witnessed many Ebola outbreaks in the past, all of which originated in Africa, in Uganda, Sudan, Zaire and other countries, but why has there been no movement in regard to prevention of further outbreaks, why has there been no advance in research for vaccination or treatment for Ebola?

The development of international organizations and global health actors was introduced as a means of solving the problems faced by traders and merchants due to health-related issues faced when national policies were the way to face infectious diseases which cross borders, in other words, health improvement has always been a by-product of economic benefits and not the priority, some scholars even argue that WHO was the fruit of the merchants pushing on their governments (Fidler, D. P., 2001). so is the reaction late because of the lack of incentives and undermining of its effect on the global north?

In this epidemic the first cases were recorded in Guinea in December 2013 and then it started spreading to Liberia and Sierra Leone (Periods, K. T. 2014), while the first roadmap set by global actors was published in August 2014, eight months after the cases recorded in Guinea, which shows a clear belated response to the emergency. The fact that the efforts on global level are belated hinders the successful international cooperation, a factor -amog others- that led to the relatively huge spread of such a disease (Fidler, D. P., 2001).

Ebola is currently a living example indicating Global governance malfunction, which signifies the need to face the problems of the framework upon which global health governance can be built, and the need to define leadership and authority. Of course economic barriers and resources are the major issues to be solved -for what the director general of WHO mentioned about cutting its budget, which had an effect on emergency response department in the organization- and by definition, how can states work together in a cohesive way to achieve the results aimed at (Dodgson R. Lee, K. and Drager, N., 2002).

Ebola, Health and Health systems

Ebola can be fought by the immune system of humans' body, yet the effective response is delayed –Hypersensitivity reaction type 4- and takes a few weeks to develop. A functioning immune system needs good general health in order to respond, and this is related to other determinants of health like nutrition and general fitness. Poverty rate in Sierra Leone is 52.9% (WBD, 2014). On top of that comes illiteracy and cultural behaviors which together create a good environment for Ebola to spread and make management of patients more difficult(Farmer, P., 2008).

When conditions above are combined with anemic healthcare system in Sierra Leone, such a disease –although not highly contagious- cant be controlled or managed properly. Ebola, until today, has no cure and its management is only supportive, which means patients are treated symptomatically until their body is capable of fighting the disease, in Sierra Leone there are 2 nurses per 10,000, of course less physicians - due to brain drain-, and distant health facilities makes this supportive management not expected to be delivered, or at least not in a proper way (World bank database, 2014). This shows the gap in global governance and the poor prediction of and prevention of such disasters. Ebola is a lesson for the future – because due to globalization and interconnectedness of the world, diseases don't know borders anymore –, healthcare systems must be strengthened globally to be able to cope up with such disasters and prevent outbreaks (Fryatt, R., Mills, A., & Nordstrom, A., 2010). A clear example of the capability of proper healthcare systems to contain outbreaks is the US system, one case was diagnosed, two locally infected but no further spread, on the contrary, more than 9,000 have been affected in Africa with a mortality rate of approximately 50 % (CDC, 2014).

Realistically, this cant be done by each state alone, or public sectors alone, as huge amounts of money should be shifted to meet the needs of strengthening healthcare systems, so it must be a collaborative work on different levels, national and global, public and private, all must contribute to this goal (Fryatt, R., Mills, A., & Nordstrom, A., 2010). At Alma-Ata it was agreed globally on the principle of health as a human right and the concept of Primary Health Care which basically aimed at improving healthcare systems in states, funds were raised for that purpose and the world had one vision (Chan, M., 2008), yet with the emergence of the World Bank as a global power, and some of the international health actors, WHO started to have diminished role in terms of leading the world health. Recommendations from the world Bank –which was clearly against Alma-Ata outcomes (Lister and Labonte, 2009) –to privatize health service provision was adopted by most of the countries, and the shift from strengthening the health systems to vertical programs, which led to stasis of health systems with no or slight improvement. The world –

especially the poor –are facing the consequences of such recommendations as Ebola currently shows (Brugha, R., & Zwi, A., 2002).

Ebola and the work of organizations

Globally, there have been generous donations from countries like Canada, Australia, America and the EU, as from other organizations like the WHO, UN and WB. Donations are estimated to be in billions of dollars to affected countries, yet is money is the only issue? MSF has sent its volunteer doctors to work on field in affected countries.

On national level, government in Sierra Leone instituted new protocols at the International Airport, It also restricted public and other mass gatherings, quarantine measures for communities affected by Ebola were made; travel in and out of those communities will be restricted until a medical team clears them. Authorized house-to-house searches to locate and quarantine Ebola patients and requires all deaths be reported before burial. Lastly authorized police and military personnel to help enforce these and other prevention and control measures and required local government officials to establish laws to support Ebola prevention efforts (CDC, 2014). According to WB, if the Ebola epidemic is contained by the end of 2014, the economic impacts on West Africa, including on Guinea, Liberia and Sierra Leone, could be lessened and economies would

begin to recover and catch up quickly. If the crisis continues into 2015 as predicted, slower growth could cost the region $32.6 billion over 2014 and 2015 and lead to much higher levels of poverty.

Civil society organizations have been working in collaboration with MSF and other NGOs, yet not formally engaged by the government, active involvement of civil society and international NGOs can improve the progress of management of the epidemic (Edwards, M., 2009).

Pharmaceutical companies and research institutes must also take an active part in future prevention of such epidemics, as mentioned before there were multiple outbreaks of Ebola before, starting in 1976 yet until now no cure or vaccine is available. Is it because of the nature of the virus? Or is it because of the expected financial loses to be invested and incentives to be lacking in a disease which is almost confined to poor populations of the world? Hopefully this epidemic will change that concept and more researches are to be done to fight Ebola. Developing world, although not rich in resources or equipments, needs to invest in science in a way that is balanced to narrow the global technology gap between the two poles of the world, thus it must be in a way that it serves the public population needs (Acharya, T., 2007).

The way forward...

As mentioned above, the Ebola is not an epidemic candidate due to its pathology and virus nature, yet this has turned to an epidemic due to the global pathology. This epidemic will take its time to kill people, but it will come to end soon because humans are not carriers for the virus. But what has the world learnt from it?

Ebola has identified the defect within the global health leadership. A proposed solution to the global health challenges is the reform of WHO as a global health leader, which should be the legalizing and main decision maker on global level, not an advisory or technical body as it is now. In further details, the WHO is to take the roles of global stewardship, a leadership role in setting global health norms and be the support provider to countries, and of course coordinate the work of the many global health actors to assure better outcomes, and lastly is its unique role in governance being the major global *intergovernmental* health organization, WHO has a unique convening power and mandate for decision-making on major health-related issues (*Moon, S., Szlezák, N. A., Michaud, C. M., Jamison, D. T., Keusch, G. T., Clark, W. C., & Bloom, B. R., 2010*).

Of course, such a reform will be hard to implement due to the many different global actors and different incentives and motives behind each organization, taking for example three different actors to see the suspected arguments of such a move and putting their arguments in mind bridge the gap in between.

The first actor would be the WHO itself, to whom the advantages will be numerous, as it would take the leadership role back as it used to be when created, it would also have more

financial support and more freedom of expenditure along to its priorities, it would also organize the work of other nongovernmental organizations worldwide. On the other hand this might be a huge power to one actor, and with more power comes bigger responsibilities. it also raise the expectations towards the outcomes organized by it, putting it more under the global microscope. Such authority will make it the body to blame when things go out of control, but with better understanding, rational decision making and cost effective measures such obstacles can be overcome.

From another global actor aspect like the world bank's, which has gained more power due to its economic power, it will be beneficial as it would take the responsibilities of global health problems incurred by their decisions and be less under focus in global health problems; yet this means there will be a shift of power to another actor, who might influence the decisions taken by the WB and hinder -in an economic way- their health-related economy control.

The other groups of actors, taking Doctors without Borders as an example for nongovernmental organizations, would benefit from such a reform in enhancing their decisions and actions globally when passed by the WHO - as in the proposal, all actors will be united under the WHO-, which would mean more support at different levels. Disadvantages of such a reform for this type of organizations would be the lack of autonomy in some situations as all decisions would be taken by one body and inability to go against a decision passed by WHO -that in the proposal are to be implemented by the states.

These advantages and disadvantages to each different set of organizations must be weighted for the enhancement of GHG and health globally in general. This reform can be implemented by making clear definition for what GHG is, clear job description for each actor globally and clear decision-making process in a way that makes the interdependence of these different actors acknowledged, yet populations health is not to be a second priority or a victim of another global measures.

References

Acharya, T. (2007). Science and technology for wealth and health in DEVELOPING countries. Global public health, 2(1), 53-63.

Achenbach, J. (2014, 06.10.2014). Paul Farmer on Ebola: "This isn't a natural disaster, this is the terrorism of poverty", The Washington Post http://www.washingtonpost.com/blogs/achenblog/wp/2014/10/06/paul-farmer-on-ebola-this-isnt-a-natural-disaster-this-is-the-terrorism -Of - poverty/?utm_content=buffer5d498&utm_medium=social&utm_source=facebook.com&utm_campaign=buffe

Blas, E., Gilson, L., Kelly, M. P., Labonté, R., Lapitan, J., Muntaner, C., ... & Vaghri, Z. (2008). Addressing social determinants of health inequities: what can the state and civil society do?. The Lancet, 372(9650), 1684-1689.

Brugha, R., & Zwi, A. (2002). Global approaches to private sector provision: where is the evidence. Health Policy in a Globalising World. Kelley Lee and B. a. SF Kent. Cambridge, Cambridge University Press, 63-77.

CDC, 2014. Center for Disease control, USA, available at: http://cdc.gov

Chan, M. (2008). Return to Alma-Ata. The Lancet, 372(9642), 865-866.

Dodgsen R., Lee, K. and Drager, N. (2002). Global Health Governance; a conceptual review. Discussion paper No. 1. WHO & LSHTM.

Edwards, M. (2009). Civil society. Polity.

Farmer, P. (2008). Challenging orthodoxies: the road ahead for health and human rights. health and human rights, 5-19.

Fidler, D. P. (2001). The globalization of public health: the first 100 years of international health diplomacy. Bulletin of the World Health Organization, 79(9), 842-849.

Frenk, J., Gómez-Dantés, O., & Moon, S. (2014). From sovereignty to solidarity: a renewed concept of global health for an era of complex interdependence. The Lancet, 383(9911), 94-97.

Fryatt, R., Mills, A., & Nordstrom, A. (2010). Financing of health systems to achieve the health Millennium Development Goals in low-income countries. The Lancet, 375(9712), 419-426.

Gostin, L. O., & Friedman, E. A. (2014). Ebola: a crisis in global health leadership. The Lancet, 384(9951), 1323-1325.

Held, D. (2008). Global challenges: Accountability and effectiveness. a progressive agenda for global action, 23.

Lister and Labonte (2009). Chapter 8: Globalization and health system change. In Labonte R. et al (eds). Pathways, evidence and policy. New York. Pp 181-212. Routledge.

Moon, S., Szlezák, N. A., Michaud, C. M., Jamison, D. T., Keusch, G. T., Clark, W. C., & Bloom, B. R. (2010). The global health system: lessons for a stronger institutional framework. PLoS medicine, 7(1), e1000193.

Periods, K. T. (2014). Ebola virus disease in west Africa—the first 9 months of the epidemic and forward projections.

PHMS (2014). Ebola epidemic exposes the pathology of the global economic and political system. Retrieved September 14, 2014, from http://www.phmovement.org/sites/www.phmovement.org/files/phm_ebola_23_09_2014final_0.pdf

 Sifferlin A (2014), World Bank: Ebola's Economic Impact Could Be 'Catastrophic', Time, Sept. 17, 2014.
Available at: http://time.com/3394147/ebola-world-bank/

UNDP (2014). Sustaining Human progress: reducing vulnerabilities and Building resilience, Human development report. Available at: http://hdr.undp.org/sites/default/files/hdr14-summary-en.pdf

World Bank Database (2014). available at: http://worldbank.org
World population data sheet (2013).